Herbal Remedies for Sinus Infection Treatment

By Smith J. Offor

Table of Contents

Introduction

How long do sinus infections last?
There are nine ways to treat sinus infections, as well as prevention advice.

It's possible to have acute, subacute, or chronic sinusitis. These distinctions are based on how long the symptoms have lasted. Acute sinusitis typically lasts less than four weeks, subacute sinusitis lasts between four and twelve weeks sinusitis can last for up to 12 weeks if it is chronic, and it usually does.

According to a reliable source. Most sinus infections are brought on by a virus or other airborne allergen, and they usually go away on their own. A course of antibiotic therapy, however, can help bacterial sinus infections get better.

1. Drink a lot of water

For overall health, adequate hydration is crucial. A healthy body can fight infections effectively and speed up recovery if it gets enough fluids to do so.

Hydration is important for maintaining the health of the skin and mucous membranes inside the sinuses, which can be beneficial in the case of sinusitis.

lessen irritation, thin mucus, and stop further infection.

2. Rest

Most sinus infections disappear on their own in 2-3 weeks. Giving the body enough time to fight infection during this period is crucial.

Resting when you can and avoiding strenuous activity may hasten recovery.

3. Utilize a neti pot or other nasal irrigators

Often, sinusitis sufferers will use nasal irrigation to relieve their symptoms. According to research, some symptoms of persistent sinusitis can be relieved by using a neti pot and saline solution.

Observe the instructions that came with your particular neti pot. Here are some general instructions:

- The saline solution should completely fill the pot.

- 45-degree angle your head over the sink.

- Put the pot's spout inside your top nostril. Give that nostril a careful pour of the saline solution

- With the other nostril, repeat the procedure

- Make sure to clean your neti pot thoroughly after each use, and only use distilled water. Your condition could get worse if you drink water straight from the sink because it could contain contaminants like bacteria or parasites

Other kinds of nasal irrigators come in a variety of sizes and shapes and offer the same advantages.

4. Continue to hydrate your sinuses

It can be a relief to keep your sinuses hydrated. Here are some recommendations for keeping your sinuses hydrated:

- For relief from nasal blockages at night, sleep with a humidifier on in your bedroom.
- Use natural saline nasal sprays in the morning and before going to bed.
- To relieve swelling and congestion, take hot showers or use steam rooms.

5. Eat foods that naturally fight bacteria

The body's defenses against infection may be strengthened by including natural antibiotics like honey, ginger, and garlic in your meals.

Some foods also have anti-inflammatory properties, which may help reduce sinus infection swelling. Berries, leafy greens, and oily fish are a few of these.

However, there is little research on using diet changes directly to treat sinus infections, and anecdotal evidence is frequently used as support.

6. Utilize oils to clear the sinuses

Some people contend that applying essential oils topically and inhaling them can help reduce sinus congestion symptoms. For instance, a study on in vitro tissue hypothesized that the primary component of eucalyptus oil, 1,8-cineole, could reduce inflammation in human tissues.

 To determine the effectiveness of these oils in cases involving humans, more investigation is required.

People frequently apply oil topically to the chest or temples to treat sinus or upper respiratory infections, or they add it to boiling water and use a diffuser to inhale the steam to relieve symptoms. Make sure to only use food-grade essential oils. After applying one drop of each oil to the roof of your mouth, sip some water.

Since inhalation can irritate the airways and possibly exacerbate symptoms, it's crucial to only use essential oils as instructed.

7. Use warm compresses to relieve facial pain

Warm compresses may provide relief from general sinus congestion pain.

Although applying a warm, damp towel to the nose, cheeks, and eyes will not cure the infection itself, it can encourage the drainage of nasal secretions and ease symptomsTrusted Source.

8. Utilize over-the-counter (OTC) medications

Ask your pharmacist to suggest an over-the-counter medication if home remedies are not providing you with relief.

By constricting the blood vessels, over-the-counter decongestants like pseudoephedrine (Sudafed) can ease the symptoms of sinusitis. Inflammation and swelling are decreased as a result. It might facilitate sinus drainage.

Before taking pseudoephedrine, talk to your doctor or pharmacist if you have high blood pressure. For those with high blood pressure, a brand called Coricidin HBP offers a selection of cough and sinus medications.

Children should not take these medications, though.

Only follow the explicit instructions when taking decongestants.

Additional over-the-counter drugs for treating generalized sinus pain include:

- aspirin.
- Tylenol contains acetaminophen.
- Ibuprofen (Motrin, Advil).

Antihistamines may help reduce swelling if an allergic reaction leads to nasal congestion.

When taking over-the-counter medications, always heed the prescription's directions and the advice of your pharmacist.

9. Obtain a prescription

In cases of bacterial sinus infections or chronic sinusitis, doctors may advise antibiotic use. Whether a virus or bacteria is to blame for your sinus infection will be determined by your primary care physician. They'll carry it out by:

- enquiring about your symptoms
- performing a medical examination
- rubbing the inside of your nose (not a common practice)

A popular prescription medication for severe sinus infections is amoxicillin (Amoxil). A bacterial sinus infection is frequently treated with the antibiotic combination Augmentin (amoxicillin-clavulanate). Those who are allergic to penicillin, however, should not take this medication; instead, a suitable substitute will be prescribed.

A person may need to take an antibiotic for up to three weeks, depending on the type that they are takingTrusted Source. As long as your doctor has prescribed antibiotics, you should take them. Even if your symptoms get better, don't stop taking them too soon because doing so can lead to antibiotic resistance.

Seeking treatment for a sinus infection

If you or someone else has: speak with your doctor.

- a temperature that is consistently higher than 38°C (100 p.c.).

- symptoms that have persisted for more than ten days.
- signs and symptoms that are getting worse.
- symptoms that are not relieved by over-the-counter medication.
- over the past year, several sinus infections.
- You might have chronic sinusitis if you experience sinus infections for eight weeks or longer or if you get them more frequently than four times annually.

These are typical reasons for chronic sinusitis.

- allergies.
- growths on the nose.
- infections of the respiratory tract.

Why do sinus infections occur?

When the tissue in the sinuses swells, a sinus infection develops. Mucus accumulates as a result, and there is discomfort and pain.

The top portion of the respiratory tract is made up of air-filled cavities called sinuses that are located in the face's skeletal structure. The nose to throat passageway of these pockets.

Trusted Source: cites a number of variables that could prevent sinus drainage.

- the widespread cold
- Itchy eyes and nose
- exposition to allergens
- air pressure shifts

The Centers for Disease Control and Prevention Source states that viruses are responsible for 90% of adult sinus infections.

In order to lower your chance of developing a sinus infection:

- Always wash your hands after being in a crowded area, such as a bus or train.
- Follow the recommended immunization schedule.
- If at all possible, avoid exposing yourself to people who have the flu or other upper respiratory infections.
- Stay away from smoking and passive smoking.
- To keep the air in your home moist, use a clean humidifier.

- To lower your risk of complications like sinusitis, get lots of sleep if you have a cold.

10 ALL-NATURAL TREATMENTS FOR SINUS INFECTIONS

What exactly is a sinus infection?
In the bones that surround the nose, there are hollow spaces called sinuses, or sinus cavities, through which air can pass. Your nasal cavities swelling and inflammation signal a sinus infection or sinusitis. Your sinuses typically contain air. Germs (bacteria, viruses, and fungi) can grow and result in an infection when sinuses become clogged and filled with fluid.

Well, that depends on what kind of sinus infection you have and how long they last. Even with proper care, acute sinusitis can persist for longer than two weeks. You're more likely to have bacterial sinusitis if your sinus infection persists for more than 10 to 14 days. Chronic sinusitis with polyps is a sinus inflammation that lasts 12 weeks or longer and is linked to nasal polyps; it lasts much longer than acute sinusitis — at least 12 weeks. Other types of chronic sinusitis also last 12 weeks or longer and are brought on by allergies or a deviated septum.

It depends on what initially caused the sinus infection to begin with, is a sinus infection contagious. You can spread a virus if it's the cause of your sinus infection. Consequently, a person who contracts your illness (the virus) will probably develop a cold, which could develop into a sinus infection but could also just be a cold. A sinus infection can occasionally result from the flu. If your sinus infection is caused by a virus, you may have been contagious days before you even noticed that you had one. A sinus infection can also be brought on by bacteria. That implies that your infection cannot spread to others. But a bacterial sinus infection typically lasts longer and is more severe than a viral sinus infection.

Your doctor will not be able to determine whether your sinus infection is viral or bacterial based solely on your symptoms or an examination. The length of the symptoms is the best indicator of the cause of a sinus infection. After five to seven days, if the sinus infection is viral, it should start to get better. On the other hand, a bacterial infection frequently persists for seven to ten days, if not longer, and it may even worsen after that time.

WHAT A SINUS INFECTION ENTAILS

Symptoms and signs

Both acute and chronic sinusitis share several symptoms that are specific to sinus infections.

- You're sneezing a thick, yellow, pungent fluid

- Obstruction in your nose

- Congestion.

- Post-nasal drip

- Surrounding your face and eyes, sinus pressure or pain

- Headache, which is frequently referred to as a "sinus headache" and typically affects the forehead

- a cold that persists or worsens

- Fatigue

- Cough

- Fever

- Earaches

It's critical to remember that each of these signs and symptoms can accompany a common cold. You could have a sinus infection if these symptoms last for more than 10 days. Acute sinusitis may be the cause if you experience two or more symptoms as well as thick, green or yellow nasal discharge.

In addition to experiencing these symptoms for 12 weeks or longer, chronic sinusitis can also cause the following symptoms:

- a feeling of congestion or heaviness in your face

- nasal mucus is present

- runny nose or postnasal drainage that is discolored

- Breath problems

- a toothache

- frequently feeling exhausted

Risk factors and causes

A sinus infection can result from any medical condition, including:

respiratory illnesses, such as the common cold.

- Hay fever or being exposed to allergens like cigarette smoke, dry air, and pollutants.

- nasal polyps, a deviated septum, or a nasal bone spur, among other obstructions in the nasal or sinus cavities.

- Non-allergic rhinitis, also known as symptoms of allergies for which there is no known cause.

- air pressure changes (caused, for instance, by swimming or ascending to high altitudes).

- bacterial infections brought on by dental issues.

- injury to the sinuses physically.

- viruses, fungi, and microbes.

- Streptococcus pneumoniae, Haemophilusinfluenzae, Moraxella catarrhalis, Staphylococcus aureus, and Streptococcus pyogenes are the five most typical bacteria that can cause sinus infections

The following list of sinus infection risk factors includes some that also serve as causes:

- suffering from asthma.
- use of nasal decongestants excessively.
- frequent diving or swimming.
- reaching high altitudes by climbing or flying.
- Nasal bone spurs, nasal polyps (minor growths or swellings in the nasal passage), or other anomalies like a deviated septum or cleft palate.
- dental disease.
- exposure to tobacco smoke and air pollution

Pregnancy
Disease caused by gastroesophageal reflux (GERD).

Being in the hospital, particularly if your illness or injury required the placement of a tube in your nose (such as a nasogastric tube from your nose to your stomach).

Treatment as is customary
If your symptoms persist for more than 10 days or if the sinus infection is determined to be bacterial, many doctors will advise antibiotics for it. You do not at all need to take antibiotics if the cause of your sinus infection is viral. A simple acute sinus infection is frequently treated with amoxicillin (Amoxil). Amoxicillin-clavulanate (Augmentin), which is said to typically be effective against most of the

species and strains of bacteria that cause bacterial sinus infections, is also frequently used by doctors as their drug of choice for treating suspected bacterial sinus infections.

Numerous medical professionals will also suggest mucolytics, antihistamines, painkillers, decongestants, anti-inflammatory drugs, and nasal corticosteroids. It's crucial to read the side effects of any prescribed medications. It's also critical to be aware that many doctors still recommend antibiotics for viral sinus infections, which only worsens the issue of antibiotic resistance.

10 All-Natural Cure for Sinus Infections

1. Suitable Foods & Drinks for Sinus Infections

Water — Staying properly hydrated is essential to eliminating the virus from your body. Drink 8 ounces or more every 2 hours, if possible.

In addition to providing essential minerals, chicken broth with vegetables is a traditional remedy for respiratory and nasal irritation.

Horseradish: Horseradish has a powerful ability to open nasal passages, as anyone who has accidentally consumed too much horseradish can attest. To make it even stronger, combine some lemon juice with horseradish.

Ginger: To hasten the healing process, make a ginger tea and add some raw honey.

Both the vegetables garlic and onions support immune system function.

Foods high in vitamin C —Eating foods high in vitamin C can strengthen the immune system and hasten sinusitis recovery.

2. Foods & Drinks to Avoid

White blood cells, which aid in infection resistance, are decreased by sugar.

Fruit juices —While orange juice does contain some vitamin C, it is not as abundant as whole fruits or vegetables in this vitamin.

Juice should be diluted before drinking.

Dairy products — Milk and other dairy products should be avoided as they tend to produce mucus.

Refined flour and grains —All refined grains have the potential to increase mucus production.

Salt: Salt can dehydrate you if you don't drink enough water, which will prolong the time it takes for your sinus inflammation to heal.

3. Oil of oregano

Carvacrol and thymol, two potent compounds found in oregano oil, have potent anti-bacterial and anti-fungal properties. I advise taking 500 mg of oregano oil four times a day. A few drops of oregano oil can also be added to a large bowl of recently boiled water to treat sinus infections. A safe distance away from the hot water, cover your head with a towel to create a tent to trap the steam inside. Close your eyes, place your face over the pot, and breathe in the fragrant steam for a few minutes. This can be done several times daily to help clear the nasal passages.

4. Extract from grapefruit seeds

Strong antiviral qualities can be found in grapefruit seed extract. For this reason, many nasal and throat sprays contain it. The primary biological components in grapefruit seeds—known as limonoids and naringenin—are thought to be in charge of the fruit's capacity to exterminate infectious invaders. (15) Four times a day, I advise using a nasal spray containing grapefruit seed extract.

5. vitamins C

The immune system, which guards against infection and aids in the body's ability to fight off an infection once it has occurred, functions properly only when vitamin C is present. Vitamin C functions as an antioxidant and aids in protecting our cells from oxidative stress. Air pollution and cigarette smoke are two examples of substances that contain free radicals and can thus frequently contribute to the development of sinus infections.

6. Garlic

The best antibiotics in nature are found in garlic. Since sinus infections frequently result from colds, garlic is a fantastic way to not only naturally treat a sinus infection but also to prevent one from developing in the first place. During the cold season (November to February), participants in one study took either garlic supplements or a placebo for 12 weeks. If they did catch a cold, those who took garlic did so less frequently than those who took a placebo, and they recovered more quickly. Over the course of the 12-week treatment period, those who didn't take garlic (the placebo group) were much more likely to catch more than one cold. According to the study, allicin, garlic's main biologically active component, is responsible for its capacity to protect against the common cold virus.

The World Health Organization suggests consuming two to five grams (or about one clove) of fresh garlic, 0 point four to one point two grams of dried garlic powder, two to five milligrams of garlic oil, 300 to 1,000 milligrams of garlic extract, or other preparations that are equivalent to two to five milligrams of allicin on a daily basis for adults to promote general health.

7. The herb echinacea

The herb echinacea can aid your body in warding off bacteria and viruses. This herb is frequently suggested by licensed herbalists as an all-natural sinus infection remedy. A sinus infection can be treated with echinacea thanks to its active ingredients, which have been proven in scientific studies to have antiviral, immune-boosting, and pain- and inflammation-reducing properties. It is best to start taking echinacea supplements as soon as symptoms appear.

8. The Neti Pot

Additionally, sinus problems can be significantly improved and the nasal passageways can be cleaned by using a neti pot and saline solution. Nasal irrigation is the name of this procedure. "Research reported in the Canadian Medical Association Journal has even demonstrated that using a neti pot can eliminate some symptoms of chronic sinusitis and maintain positive results over a six-month period.

Lead author Dr. Paul Little, a professor of medicine at the University of Southampton, claims that patients reported fewer headaches, a decrease in the use of over-the-counter medications, and a decreased likelihood of returning to the doctor for another case of sinusitis.

9. Include moisture

Adding more moisture to the air and your nasal passages—whether it's through a humidifier, saline nasal spray, or simply sitting in a steamy bathroom—can significantly lessen congestion. If you have a sinus infection, I strongly advise sleeping with a humidifier on. A natural saline nasal spray that you can buy and use as directed on the packaging several times a day is also an option. Particularly effective at lessening sinus headaches is steam inhalation.

10.   Essential oils

Using eucalyptus oil and peppermint oil can be very successful in helping to naturally clear the sinuses. These essential oils have a natural ability to clear mucus, open up the sinuses, and get rid of infections. To do this, only use food-grade essential oils and apply one drop of each to the roof of the mouth.

Drink water next.

Diffusing essential oils into the air so you can breathe them in is another fantastic idea. Sinus infections can also benefit from using my homemade vapor rub recipe.

Precautions

You should visit your doctor if your sinus infection symptoms worsen or do not go away after 10 to 14 days. Bronchitis, complications, and the need for surgery can develop from an untreated sinus infection, among other conditions.

You might also seek advice from an allergist if you initially experience symptoms that are similar to allergies because they may be able to identify the source of your symptoms.

If you are pregnant, nursing, have any ongoing health issues, or are currently taking other medications, always consult your doctor before taking any natural supplements.

Sinus infections, sadly, are fairly typical in today's society.

similarly, unneeded antibiotic therapy.

Keep in mind that treating viral sinus infections—of which the majority are caused by viruses—does not at all require the use of antibiotics. When taken when they are not truly necessary, antibiotics can cause much more harm to your body than good.

Natural treatments for sinusitis work well for the majority of sinus infections. There are so many natural options available that are not only affordable and simple to carry out in the comfort of your home, but also highly effective.

Five incredibly efficient home remedies for treating sinusitis naturally

The inflammation or swelling of the tissue lining the sinuses characterizes sinus infection, also referred to as sinusitis. The four pairs of cavities (spaces) that can be found in the head are known as sinuses. A few tiny channels connect these four cavities. These channels function as drainage, assisting in keeping the nose germ-free and clean. When these channels fill with fluid and obstruct the path in the nose, sinus infection results. Water can build up in these channels, where bacteria can flourish and lead to an infection (bacterial sinusitis).

What Leads to a Sinus Infection?

In addition to the previously mentioned factors, one of the main causes of a sinus infection is a cold, which results in sinus swelling and inflammation and causes a buildup of mucus inside the nasal passages. Snoring, breathing difficulties, particularly when sleeping or lying down, acute headaches, and in severe cases, meningitis or brain fever with severe symptoms, are just a few of the issues that this condition can cause. We understand your concern; however, despite the fact that this condition can be challenging to manage, there are some simple home remedies that are reputed to offer immediate relief when it appears to be deteriorating.

Natural Home Remedies for Sinusitis. We've got some quick and simple natural home remedies for treating sinus infections, so if you're in pain, try one of them.

Examine them quickly:

- vinegar made from apple cider.

- This amazing ingredient has a number of advantages for your health.

- ACV, also referred to as apple cider vinegar, has antibacterial properties that can be used to treat flu symptoms like a cold, cough, allergies, etc. Take a spoonful of ACV and mix it with some water to drink to get the benefits.

- Therapy using steam

- Try taking a hot shower or using the steam breathe technique to help open your nasal passages - who doesn't know how effective steam therapy is for managing cold and flu symptoms? All you have to do is take a bowl, fill it with hot water, cover your face and head with a towel, and breathe in the steam. You'll experience immediate relief from sinus infection-related congestion as a result of this instantly opening your nasal passages.

Turmeric

The most significant spice that is simple to locate in the kitchen is turmeric, which has a wealth of antioxidant properties. The best treatment for sinus symptoms is thought to be turmeric. Additionally, this spice has anti-inflammatory qualities that aid in easing sinusitis symptoms. Simply mix a small amount of turmeric into your hot tea and drink it. This will assist in clearing out the mucus that has built up in the channels and open up the nasal passages.

Essential oil of eucalyptus

This essential oil improves respiratory health while being excellent at treating sinus infections. You only need to breathe in a few drops of eucalyptus oil that have been placed in a handkerchief. Your nasal congestion will disappear right away thanks to this. For best results, use it daily.

The cayenne pepper

One of the most potent spices for treating sinusitis at home, cayenne powder is thought to be effective when used correctly. It can unclog blocked nasal passageways and clear sinuses. All you have to do is thoroughly stir the cayenne powder into a glass of water, preferably hot. Now, consume this two to three times per day. Add some honey as well, if you'd like. However, you shouldn't consume this mixture if you have a mouth ulcer.

What natural remedies can relieve sinus pressure?

Although a person can treat sinus pressure with medication, natural remedies like saline irrigation and steam inhalation may also help to reduce symptoms and hasten the healing process.

The sinuses are lined with a type of skin called mucous membrane. By creating mucus, which traps debris and other irritants that could otherwise make the body sick, this membrane defends the body.

If someone has an allergic reaction or an infection, their sinus lining may swell.

Pressure may be felt above the eyes, on the cheeks, and around the nose as a result of swelling.

It might hurt or feel tender in these facial regions.

Uncomfortable sinus pressure may result from infections or allergies. This symptom may be lessened by blowing one's nose.

The natural remedies for sinus pressure listed below are an alternative to over-the-counter (OTC) medications.

Nostril sprays.
Steroid nasal sprays can aid in reducing nasal passageway inflammation. Many of these sprays are over-the-counter (OTC).

Other home remedies for treating sinus pressure include decongestant and saline nasal sprays.

In order to choose a nasal spray that won't interact with their medications or condition, people who have preexisting conditions like high blood pressure should speak with a doctor.

Vaporizers and humidifiers
The mucous membranes and sinuses can become dry and irritated by dry air.

The arid air will make the irritation and sinus pressure worse, despite the fact that drying out extra mucus might seem like a good idea.

Water is introduced into the air by humidifiers and vaporizers. The moisturizing
45

effects of the humid air on the delicate skin lining the sinuses are enhanced by breathing it inBoth devices exude moisture, but they do so in slightly different ways: A humidifier blows out cool, moist vapor, whereas a vaporizer warms the water to exude a warm mist.

In bedrooms and other areas where people spend a lot of time, the increased humidity is especially beneficial. One of these devices running while you sleep can help relieve sinus pressure and may help you wake up with less congestion.

The neti pot
Some people rinse their noses with neti pots, which relieve sinus pressure and keep the

mucous membranes moist. The apparatus has a long spout that resembles a small pot.

Using a neti pot involves:

- cleaning one's hands.
- by adding sterile water to the pot.
- standing directly over a sink.
- the sideways head tilt.
- gently inserting the spout into the highest nostril.
- mouth-breathing is mouth-breathing.

water being poured into the nostril
Water will flow from one nostril to the other, clearing pollen, bacteria, and other particles from the air. This procedure should be carried out on both nostrils.

It is crucial that people use sterile or distilled water instead of tap water, which can be purchased at a drugstore. Water can also be heated and then allowed to cool.

watering with salt

Nasal irrigation with saline solution can help lessen nasal irritation and inflammation.

With sterile water, salt, and baking soda, you can quickly create a saline solution at home. Mix the following ingredients together.

- quarter pint of pure water.

- one-fourth of a teaspoon (tsp) of salt.

- Baking soda, 1/4 teaspoon.

- One nostril at a time, people can inhale this from cupped palms. A syringe can also be used to inject a liquid into somconc's nostrils

breathing in steam

People can easily practice steam inhalation at home. Lean over so that the face is directly over the water after boiling water has been poured into a big bowl. Breathe through the nose while wearing a towel over the head.

Directly breathing over a steaming kettle or boiling pot of water is not advised. Skin can be burned by the steam.

Showers and baths.

Instead of boiling water, one can simply turn on the shower. Steam from hot baths and showers can easily fill a space. A person's sinus passages become more moist when they breathe in this steam, which also helps to moisturize the surrounding air.

The additional moisture can reduce sinusitis and thin out mucus to make sinus clearing simpler.

Acupressure.
Applying pressure to particular body points with acupressure helps to reduce pain and other ill-effects by relieving tension. Acupressure may alleviate some symptoms, but scientists are unsure if it actually relieves symptoms.

Acupressure is frequently credited with being able to treat sinus issues, various flus, and colds.

Acupressure can be practiced at home or by visiting a professional.

Hydration.
Maintaining body hydration is crucial whenever someone is ill.

The nasal passages' mucous membranes can remain moist and function properly with the help of proper hydration.

While all liquids can aid in hydration, The 2020–2025 Dietary Guidelines for Americans advise people to give plain water and unflavored juices a higher priority when consuming liquids.

compression using a hot washcloth.

Pressure can also be reduced by applying heat to the sinus region. Using a warm washcloth is one of the simplest ways to accomplish this.

Wring out a clean washcloth after running it under water that is not too hot. For a few minutes, fold it and lay it across the cheeks and nose bridge.

Aromatic substances

Many people assert that using essential oils can help relieve sinus congestion symptoms. Essential oils are pure natural oils that are extracted from plants.

Eucalyptus and peppermint oils are frequently used to treat sinus inflammation. When using a diffuser or a steam bath, people can use these essential oils by adding a few drops.

Habits of sleep

For a number of reasons, sleep can reduce sinus pressure.

Rest is crucial to a body's ability to heal and advance the healing process. Additionally, while you are sleeping, your body makes more white blood cells. These cells are necessary for getting rid of any viruses or bacteria that might be aggravating the sinuses and raising the pressure inside them.

Sleeping while propped up may be more comfortable for someone with sinus pressure.

To do this, they can add additional pillows to the upper back or behind the head.

In order to prevent a stuffy nose from disturbing your sleep, try sleeping with your head propped up.

This may help mucus move through your sinuses and nasal passages. On the other hand, lying flat may cause more pressure and mucus to accumulate.

Nasal congestion while sleeping in this location.

With time, these natural sinus pressure relief methods can aid in symptom relief and improve breathing. However, it is crucial to avoid doing anything that could delay recovery. These comprise:

Breathing dry air: Dry air, like that found in saunas, can aggravate the sinuses and make recovery more difficult.

Chemical inhalation: On an average day, sinus irritation can be caused by cleaning products like chlorine and bleach. Those who already have inflamed sinuses may find that they make them worse.

Blowing too forcefully: If someone's sinuses feel blocked, they may try to blowing their nose to try and get some of the mucus out. People should be careful not to blow too forcefully. Pressure that is applied too heavily can hurt and even make pressure worse.

Increasing sinus pressure after flying is a common side effect for people who are ill and flying. After landing, the majority of sinus pressure from flying will subside within a few hours. However, because their sinuses are already irritated, people who fly may experience even more sinus pressure from the flight if they have an upper respiratory infection or sinus infection. It is advised to change the flight until the infection clears.

How does sinus pressure look in the future?

If an infection, like sinusitis, is to blame, the pressure should subside within a few weeks.

Sinus pressure may fluctuate if an allergy is to blame. When an allergen, such as grass or pet fur, is encountered beforehand, sinus pressure can be avoided by taking antihistamines.

The natural treatments mentioned above can aid in easing sinus discomfort and pressure.

They may also hasten the healing process.

Home remedies, however, might not always be effective.

People should see a doctor if they haven't recovered from an infection after using home remedies.

how to activate the sinus pressure points.

It may help to relieve nasal congestion or a stuffy nose to stimulate pressure points in the sinuses. It entails locating specific pressure points close to the nose and using circular fingertip motions to apply pressure to those areas.

Although there are many remedies for stuffy noses, including pills and nasal sprays, they can have side effects. This might prompt someone to search for complementary or alternative strategies to relieve congestion.

In this piece, we examine sinus pressure points—what they are, where they are, and how to activate them.

- Infographic.
- Diego Sabogal's artwork.

Sinus pressure points: what are they?
As a component of traditional Chinese medicine, acupuncture is where the concept of pressure points originated. In acupuncture, specialists use tiny needles to stimulate particular body points. The goal is to move stagnant Qi, or vital energy, around.

Acupressure is a non-invasive technique that one can try at home that stimulates these points without the use of needles. Some claim that activating the sinus pressure points relieves their nasal congestion.

What location are they in?

The primary pressure points in the face that may relieve sinus pain or congestion are noted by the Acupuncture Association of Chartered Physiotherapists.

Each point's names, locations, and advantages are listed in the table below. A person's "body inch," as it is known to acupuncturists, is the distance between the two joints of the middle finger.

Name of the point Location Advantage

Nasal congestion, jaw problems, and paralysis of the facial muscles are all symptoms of LI19, which is located halfway between the bottom of the nostril and the lip.

Nasal congestion, respiratory issues, and facial swelling are all symptoms of LI20 0.5 cun to the side of the nostril groove.

When the eyes are forward-facing, ST3 should be level with the lower edge of the nostril and parallel to the pupil. This position also corresponds to sinus pain, dental pain, and facial muscle paralysis.

sinus issues and frontal headaches are EX-HN 3 symptoms in the middle of the brow ridge.

With general headaches, another point, GV23, might also be helpful. One cun behind the hairline, in the middle of the forehead, is where it can be found.

Activating pressure points

When practicing acupressure, a person will self-massage particular pressure points. According to the University of California, Los Angeles (UCLA), beginners should follow these steps.

- Close your eyes, unwind, and take a few deep breaths.
- Pick a pressure point and apply firm pressure with your finger.
- For several minutes, move the finger in circles or up and down.
- Press firmly and deeply.

As often as necessary, repeat this.

A person can also request that someone else massage their pressure points. The technique might produce better outcomes if you use it frequently.

UCLA advise using acupressure under a doctor's guidance.

It shouldn't hurt to stimulate pressure points.

In that case, either lower the pressure or stop the massage.

Discover additional massage methods that can facilitate sinus drainage.

Stimulation of the sinus pressure point is effective?

The effectiveness of acupressure for sinus conditions has not been thoroughly studied. Instead, a lot of studies in this field concentrate on conventional acupuncture.

For instance, in a small study published in the American Journal of Rhinology and

Allergy in 2009, researchers found that traditional acupuncture significantly reduced nasal symptoms when compared to a placebo version of the same treatment.

When to consult a doctor

While acupressure can ease nasal symptoms, some sinus conditions call for medical attention. If someone experiences: they ought to talk to a doctor.

- persistent discomfort in the forehead, eyes, or nose.
- swelling or fever are indicators of an infection.
- breathing through the nose is challenging.

Summary

Acupressure involves stimulating specific points on the body with massage. It is different from acupuncture, which involves using needles.

A person can practice acupressure on themselves, and some find that it helps relieve nasal congestion and make breathing easier.

The effectiveness of acupressure as a sinus condition treatment still requires further scientific verification. Anecdotal evidence, however, points to a low risk of side effects and the potential to help manage the symptoms.

Anyone who experiences recurring pain or signs of infection, such as fever or swelling, should see a doctor.

Alternative and complementary medicine for ear, nose, and throatHeadache and migraines.

Treatments and natural remedies for sinus infections.

Antibiotics, nasal decongestants, oral steroids, and antifungal medications are among the potential medical remedies for sinus infections. Nasal irrigation, steam inhalation, and over-the-counter analgesics are a few examples of home remedies.

The sinuses are air-filled cavities that encircle the nose. Ethmoid sinuses are located between the eyes. Middle of the head is where the sphenoids are located. Excess mucus that blocks the sinuses leads to a sinus infection.

Mucus from the nose easily drains when the sinuses are clear, removing dirt and bacteria. A sinus infection happens when too much mucus accumulates in the sinuses, creating an environment that is moist and stagnant and ideal for viruses, bacteria, or fungi to grow.

Runny or stuffy nose, pain or pressure in the face, and sore throat are just a few of the signs of a sinus infection. Sinusitis is another term for a sinus infection.

Domestic remedies

To help prevent antibiotic resistance, the ACAAI advises that people only attempt antibiotic treatment for a sinus infection if symptoms last longer than 7 to 10 days.

The following home remedies may help people with sinus infection symptoms.

prescription and over-the-counter painkillers.

Painkillers sold over-the-counter (OTC) may be used to treat sinus infection symptoms.

Some examples of these drugs are:

- only adults over the age of 18 should take aspirin.
- acetaminophen, found in medications like Tylenol.
- Advil or Motrin contain ibuprofen.
- Localized pain, fever, and headaches are just a few symptoms that OTC painkillers may help with.
- sprays for the nose.

OTC decongestant nasal sprays should only be used for a short period of time, no more than three to four days. Saline and steroid nasal sprays, for example, are OTC nasal sprays that can be used for a longer period of time. As mucus can drain from the sinuses, nasal sprays may help to lessen nasal passage swelling.

When using nasal decongestant sprays, people must use caution. The nasal passages may swell and close up as a result of rebound phenomenon, which can be brought on by excessive nasal spray use.

To prevent any negative side effects, it's crucial to carefully adhere to product instructions.

It is best to consult a doctor before using nasal sprays if a person has an existing medical condition or is pregnant.

Irrigating the nose.
The signs of a sinus infection might be lessened with nasal irrigation. In a 2016 study, it was discovered that nasal irrigation users experienced fewer headaches, fewer symptoms, and a lower need for over-the-counter medications.

In order to rinse their noses, people can use either a rinse bottle or a neti pot, a tiny container with a spout. Using a neti pot with the incorrect kind of water can be risky.

It's crucial to avoid filling a neti pot directly from the faucet. Stomach acid destroys any bacteria or parasites present, making tap water safe to drink. Using a neti pot with tap water could result in a serious infection since the nasal environment cannot kill these kinds of germs.

It is suggested that users follow one of the following precautions in order to use a neti pot safely:

- Before using, boil tap water for three to five minutes.
- putting any previously boiled water in a clean, sealed container and using it within 24 hours.
- buying water that has been sterilized or distilled.
- water is filtered using a unique, harmful-organism-trapping filter.

To use with a nasal bulb, syringe, or neti pot, people can prepare their own irrigation solution. The American Academy of Allergy, Asthma, and Immunology (AAAAI) advises using the following remedy and technique to irrigate the nose.

- Mix three teaspoons (tsp) of iodide-free salt with one teaspoon (tsp) of baking soda using a clean, airtight container and spoon.
- To one cup, or eight ounces (oz), of sterile water, add one teaspoon of the salt and baking soda mixture.
- Reduce the dry mixture quantity if the solution causes any stinging or burning sensations.
- Use one-half teaspoon of the dry mixture and four ounces of water when making the solution for kids.

- Apply the solution with a tiny syringe or a neti pot.

- Rotate the head to the left over a sink and while breathing through the mouth, gently squeeze 4 ounces of the saline rinse into the right nostril.

- Turn your head to the right and repeat on the other side after the solution has been rinsed out of your left nostril.

- After use, rinse with sterile water and completely dry the neti pot or syringe.

Breathing in steam

Even though there isn't enough data to support it, some people may find that inhaling steam helps them feel better.

One can lean over a bowl of hot water and cover their head with a towel to contain the steam to use steam inhalation to relieve sinus infection symptoms. They are able to do this for 10 to 15 minutes, three to four times daily.

One or two drops of an essential oil, like peppermint or eucalyptus oil, may be added to the water. The anti-inflammatory and antibacterial qualities of eucalyptus oil may aid in the fight against the infection.

Both health food stores and online retailers sell eucalyptus essential oil.

Rest

While suffering from a sinus infection, people should try to get lots of rest. By doing so, the body will be able to heal and focus its energy on battling the infection.

Resting and remaining at home can also aid in limiting the spread of the infection.

Hydration

During a sinus infection, drinking plenty of clear liquids will help the body stay hydrated. The recommended daily water intake for people is several glasses.

Other than soda or coffee, any liquid can be helpful. When suffering from a sinus infection, people should drink, for instance:

- transparent liquid.
- honey, ginger, or hot water with lemon.

- Herbal brews.

- Broth.

- use warm compresses

The pain and pressure caused by the clogged sinuses may be reduced by placing a warm compress on your face.

People can make a warm compress by soaking a clean facecloth in hot water, wringing it out, and applying it to the face's trouble spots, like the nose and forehead.

Antihistamines

Antihistamines aid in the management of allergic reaction-related inflammation. Because of this, they might be successful in treating sinus infections that cause symptoms similar to those of a sinus infection, like reducing sinus and nasal swelling.

OTC combination medications

Antihistamines and decongestants may be included in some over-the-counter medications. Before using these, people should consult a pharmacist or doctor because they might dry out and thicken mucus rather than loosen it.

Treatments

If home remedies for sinus infections have failed, medical treatments aim to unblock and drain the sinuses.

Antibiotics

Sinus infections MostTrusted Source get better without antibiotics.

An antibiotic prescription may be given, in accordance with the ACAAI, if a person has had a bacterial sinus infection for more than 7 to 10 days.

Two weeks may be enough time for viral sinus infections to heal.

Nasal spray on prescription

A prescription nasal spray may help lessen nasal passage swelling if over-the-counter remedies are ineffective. By doing this, mucus from the sinuses can drain more easily.

A saline solution may also be recommended by a physician to help clear excess nasal mucus.

A doctor may recommend compounded irrigation solutions containing steroids or antibiotics for chronic sinusitis.

Orally administered steroids

A doctor might recommend oral steroids for severe or persistent sinusitis. These are potent medications, so patients should first discuss any potential side effects with their doctor.

Surgery

A person might require surgery to clear the blocked sinuses and restore normal mucus drainage if a sinus infection does not improve with medication or other treatments, or if the infection has spread.

Anti-fungal drugs

A doctor might recommend antifungal medication if a fungal infection is the root of your sinusitis.

For most people, surgical treatment is also necessary to get the fungus out of their sinuses.

Symptoms

The following are signs of a sinus infection:

- clogged nose.
- altered ability to smell.
- due to post-nasal drainage, there is extra mucus in the throat
- headache
- Experiencing pain or pressure in the face
- coughing

- an aching throat

- an illness

- a bad breath

- tiredness

- teeth pain or a sore jaw

What exactly is a sinus infection?

A bacterial infection that causes your sinuses to swell up frequently results in sinus infections (also known as sinusitis). Nasal irrigation, steam therapy, drinking lots of water, using warm compresses, resting with your head elevated, and using humidifiers are a few home treatments and remedies you can try.

The most common bacterial infection that results in sinus swelling is the cause of sinus infections (sinusitis).

Nasal irrigation, steam therapy, drinking a lot of water, applying warm compresses, resting, sleeping on your side, and using humidifiers are some of the home remedies and treatments you can try.

Your sinuses will swell up if you have a sinus infection, also known as sinusitis. Symptoms of the inflamed sinuses, which resemble those of a cold, can occur. In fact, a sinus infection is frequently brought on by a cold or the flu.

Although viruses and fungi can also cause sinus infections, bacterial infections are typically to blame. These infections can be either acute or chronic. While chronic sinusitis can last for up to 12 weeks or longer, acute infections typically go away in two to three weeks.

A layer of mucus covers your sinus cavities, which helps to keep contaminants like dust and germs in check. A viral infection, such as sinusitis or a cold, can cause the lining to become inflamed and swell. Due to the sinuses' inability to drain normally, this swelling causes mucus to become stuck. When this occurs, bacteria and fungi may begin to grow in the obstructed fluid, which will result in a sinus infection.

The following are typical sinusitis signs and symptoms

- Around the cheeks, forehead, and eyes there is pressure, pain, and tenderness.

- headache brought on by the sinuses.

- nasal obstruction.

- a bad breath

- impaired taste and smell perception.

- Toothache.
- a mucous-producing cough.
- nasal mucus that is yellow or green in color
- Fever
- Fatigue
- tissue in the nose swelling
- Redness

Anyone can develop sinus infections, particularly after recovering from a cold when your defenses are weakened. However, some individuals, such as: may be more vulnerable to developing them.

- people whose sinus openings are narrow.
- individuals who have nasal polyps.
- those who suffer from a nasal bone deformity.

- allergy sufferers.

- immune system-compromised individuals.

Sinus infection treatments

For sinus infections, there are a number of natural cures and treatments you can try.

Domestic remedies

Irrigation of the nose. Flushing out your nasal passages can be done with a Neti pot or a tiny bulb syringe. It may be possible to get rid of sinus mucus by gargling with a saltwater solution. This is among the best at-home remedies for sinus infections.

Steam treatment

To help clear your sinuses, try taking a hot shower and inhaling the steam. Additionally, you can inhale steam by placing your face over a bowl or pot filled with hot water. To keep the steam in, drape a towel across your shoulders.

Have some water. Drinking more water helps to thin out the mucus, which makes it an excellent home remedy for sinusitis. Stick to juice or water and try to stay away from alcohol and caffeine.

heated compress. Applying a warm compress to your face can also be a successful at-home remedy for sinus pain and pressure.

Rest

Getting some rest is one of the most crucial things you can do if you have a sinus infection. This aids your body's ability to combat the infection and hastens your recovery.

A raised bed for sleeping

Elevate your head with additional pillows while you rest or sleep. This will lessen the likelihood of the mucus becoming lodged in your sinuses at night.

Make use of a humidifier. Increase the air's humidity, especially where you sleep. Your congestion may be relieved by doing this.

Medications

You can also try a few over-the-counter (OTC) medicines to help relieve your symptoms.

nasal spray made of salt. Along with easing congestion and inflammation, this prevents your sinuses from drying out. When allergies are the problem, steroid nasal sprays can reduce congestion and inflammation.

Decongestants

Mucus can be removed by taking a decongestant.

Antibiotics

If bacteria are to blame for your sinus infection, your doctor might advise taking antibiotics to help fight the infection.

Risks associated with treatments

Use of decongestant medications, such as nasal sprays, should last no longer than three days. If you keep using it after this period of time, your congestion might get worse.

When you have sinusitis, you will probably be blowing your nose quite a bit. To prevent irritating the nasal passages and pushing bacteria higher into your sinuses, gently blow into one nostril at a time.

herbal remedies for the sinuses
Sinusitis, another name for a sinus infection, can be extremely painful and incapacitating. The common cold is the main cause of sinus infections. Allergies, ear infections, structural abnormalities, and bacterial infections (like Helicobacter pylori) are some additional triggers. Look for a fungal or dental infection if the infection has persisted for a long time.

Holistic Perspective:
Sinus infections are poorly managed by antibiotics. I have observed many doctors advising their patients to use neti pots because of this.

Herbs, essential oils, and neti pots can all be useful for treating sinusitis.

It is very beneficial to use herbs that thin mucus, fight infection, soothe tissues, and promote expectoration.

The following are herbs for the sinuses
The categories that aid in clearing and healing the sinuses are listed below. I advise using herbs topically and internally, as well as steaming with essential oils. Using these remedies at least twice a day is very beneficial.

THE EXPECTANTS ARE.

By assisting the body's production of mucus and occasionally thinning excessively thick mucus, you can aid in the movement of foreign particles up and out of the lungs.

Elecampane (Inulahelenium) and Grindelia species are herbs. (Gum weed), Balsamorhizasagittata (Balsam root), and Populus spp. Verbascumthapsus (mullein), Marrubiumvulgare (horehound), and (poplar) bud.

Essential oils: Juniperusvirgiana or Cedrusdoedara (Cedarwood), Ocimumbasilicum (Basil), Styrax benzoin (Benzoin), Citrus bergamia (Bergamot), and various eucalyptus species. , Menthapiperita (Peppermint), Santalum album (Sandalwood), Hyssopusofficinalis (Hyssop), Foeniculumvulgare (Fennel), and Commiphora spp. (Myrrh).

DECONGESTANTS:
reduce mucus production and congestion. This can lessen the likelihood of opportunistic infection.

Herbs: Ephedra nevadensis and a few other species (Mormon tea), Eriodictyoncalifornica (Yerba Santa), Urticadioica (Nettles), or Marrubiumvulgare (Horehound).

Essential oils that help with digestion include rosemary and various eucalyptus species.

Lavandulaspp, and Melaleucaalternifolia (Tea Tree). Ravinsara aromatic (Ravinsara), Menthapiperita (Peppermint), and lavender.

Reduce your intake of foods that make mucus, such as dairy, sugar, wheat, oats, barley, and rye.

DEMULCENTS:

Cover and calm down irritated or inflamed membranes to promote healing.

Herbs: Glycyrrhiza spp., Ulmusrubra, and Althea officinalis (Marshmallow). (Licorice), Plantagoovata (Plantain), and various varieties of violets. (Violet) as well as Verbascumthapsus (Mullein).

Aspects include:

Mucus membranes, for example, that are irritated or inflamed will contract, protecting them and promoting healing and recovery.

Solidago spp. (Goldenrod), the flowers and leaves of Achilleamillefolium (Yarrow), Leucanthememvulgare (Oxeye daisy), and various Ambrosia species. Salix spp., or (Ragweed). (Willow), Filipendulaulmaria (Meadowsweet), and Hamamelis spp. Myrica species, also known as "witch hazel".(Bayberry), Euphrasiaofficinalis (Eyebright), Plantago ovate (Plantain), and different species of Equisetum.(Horsetail), and Yerba mansa (Anemopsiscalifornica).

Anti-viral programs include.

Herbs: Glycyrrhiza spp., Hyssopusofficinalis, Lomatiumdissectum (Lomatium), Ligusticumporteri (Osha), Melissa officinalis (Lemon Balm), and Hyssopusofficinalis. (Licorice).

Thymus vulgaris (thyme), Rosmarinusofficinalis (rosemary), Menthapiperita (peppermint), Melaleucaalternifolia (tea tree), and various eucalyptus species are among the essential oils. Citrus bergamia (bergamot), Piper nigrum (black pepper), Melissa officinalis (lemon balm), and Hyssopusofficinalis (hyssop) are some examples.

ANTI-MICROBIALS:

Defend against microbial infection.

Herbs: Mahonia species, Hydrastiscanadensis, Allium sativum, which is used to make garlic. Balsamorhizasagittata (Balsam root), Usnea species, and (Oregon grape root) are a few examples. (Usenea), as well as different species of Populus.bud of (poplar).

The majority of essential oils are antimicrobial to at least one type of organism. Citrus bergamia (Bergamot), Juniperuscommunis (Juniper), Eucalyptus globulus (Eucalyptus), Melaleucaalternifolia (Tea Tree), Thymus vulgaris (Thyme), linalool, Pelargonium gravolens (Geranium),

Syzygiumaromaticum (Clove), and Menthapiperita (Peppermint).

The following are instructions for using a neti pot.

- 1 cup of warm, filtered or boiled water, or herbal tea, should be added to the neti pot. The water should be about as warm as the water you would use to take a shower.
- Stir in 1/4 teaspoon of sea salt, Celtic salt, rock salt, or kosher salt (DO NOT USE TABLE SALT)

You can also include:

- 20–60 drops of an herbal extract should be added to tinctures

- One teaspoon of aloe vera juice can be used to calm irritated mucous membranes.

- Put the neti pot spout in your upper nostril and allow the water to flow out of your lower nostril as you stoop over the sink with your head tilted to one side. Tilt your head forward if you experience water running down the back of your throat. The net may occasionally flow more smoothly when breathing through the mouth.

- Repeat on the other side once you've used half the pot.

- Once or twice a day, this procedure can be performed.

Formulas for the sinuses include.

INHALATION OF SINUS INFECTIOUS MATERIAL:

- 10 ml essential oil of Eucalyptus globulus (Eucalyptus).
- 10 milliliters of Melaleucaalternifolia (Tea Tree) essential oil.
- 3 milliliters of Syzygiumaromaticum (Clove) oil.
- Menthapiperita (peppermint) essential oil, 3 ml.
- 2 milliliters of linalol essential oil from thymus vulgaris (thyme).
- 2 ml of Pelargonium gravolens (Geranium) essential oil.
- Place a towel over your head and place your head over a pot of steaming (not boiling) water. Add a couple of drops of Sinus Infection Inhalation and take a

few deep breaths. Increase as necessary.

NETI POT DROPS FOR A SINUS INFECTION:

- 2 ounces of Yerba mansa (Anemopsiscalifornica) tincture.
- 2 ounces of black walnut (Juglansnigra) tincture
- 1 ounce of a tincture of goldenseal, Hydrastiscanadensis.
- 1 oz.of tincture made from stone root, Collinsoniacanadensis.
- Marshmallow (Althea officinalis) tincture, 1 oz.
- vegetable glycerin, 10 ml.
- Use a neti pot (typically 1 cup of warm saline water) and 30–60 drops of this

mixture to irrigate both nostrils. How to use a net pot is explained above.

SINUSITIS SPRAY:

- fifteen drops Mahonia spp. Tincture made from (Oregon Grape Root).
- 15 droplets of Echinacea spp. Tincture made from (Echinacea).
- 10 drops of Baptisiatinctoria (Wild indigo) tincture.
- one-half teaspoon of vegetable glycerin.
- 2 ounces of saltwater.
- bottle of sinus spray, 2 ounces.
- Shake vigorously after adding all the ingredients.
- Up to four times daily, spray sinuses and take deep breaths.

NASAL OIL FROM NASYA:

- One ounce of unroasted sesame oil.

- Eucalyptus globulus (Eucalyptus) essential oil, 6 drops.

- a total of 4 drops of Menthapiperita (peppermint) essential oil.

- Two drops of the Niaouli oil by Melaleucaquinquenervia.

To Use:

- Put a small pillow or towel rolled up under your neck as you recline on your back. Lean your head back.

- Fill each nostril with 5–10 drops of nasya oil.

- Inhale deeply, then lie down for a while to let the nasya work its magic.

- Gently rub the sinuses, nose, and nostrils.

- You can also put a drop of Nasya oil on your little finger and gently insert it into your nostril while standing or sitting.

SINUS SALTS:

- 14 cup whole salt (Real Salt works well).

- Rosemary oil, Rosmarinusofficinalis, 3 drops.

- Melaleucaalternifolia (Tea tree) essential oil, three drops.

- Eucalyptus radiata essential oil, 2 drops.

- In a blender or coffee grinder, combine all the essential oils with the salt and thoroughly blend. In a glass container with a tightly fitting lid, store. Dosage: Combine 1 cup of warm water with 1/4 teaspoon of the mixture. Use in a neti pot for allergies, colds, flu, and sinus infections. Use the net pot as described above.

THROAT SOOTHER:

- 2 ounces of Hydrastiscanadensis (Goldenseal).
- Eriodictyoncalifornica, also known as yerba santa, 2 oz.
- 1 point 5 ounces Stone root (Collinsonia Canadensis).

- Althea officinalis, also known as marshmallow, 10.5 oz.

    o ounces of Salvia officinalis (Sage).

- Baptisiatinctoria (Wild indigo): 1/4 oz.

- A quarter of an ounce of horseradish, Armoraciarusticana.

- 2 oz.of vegetable glycerin.

- Shake well after thoroughly combining all the ingredients. For a head cold or sinus infection, this tincture can be taken internally by taking 60 drops, 3-5 times per day. Put 30 to 60 drops in a cup of warm saline water to use it in a net pot to rinse the sinuses. How to use a net pot is explained above.

The description of an allergy

When a person reacts to environmental elements that are typically safe for most people, allergies can result. Allergens are these substances, which can be found in dust mites, pets, pollen, insects, ticks, mold, foods, and some medications.

The inherited propensity for allergic diseases to manifest is known as atopy.

An immune response that results in allergic inflammation can occur in atopic individuals after exposure to allergens.

The following symptoms could be brought on by this.

- allergies that affect the nose and/or eyes, causing hay fever-like rhinitis and/or conjunctivitis.
- eczematous or urticaria-prone skin.

- asthma is caused by the lsungs.

How does an allergic reaction manifest itself?

An allergic reaction happens when an allergen that a person is allergic to comes into contact with it:

- A body responds with an antibody response when an allergen (like pollen) enters the body.

- Mast cells are the site of the antibodies' attachment.

- The mast cells respond by releasing histamine when the pollen interacts with the antibodies.

- The inflammation (redness and swelling) that results when histamine is released as a result of an allergen is upsetting and uncomfortable.

Some chemicals and food additives can have comparable effects. However, they are referred to as adverse reactions rather than allergies if the immune system is not involved.

Which body parts could be impacted?

Depending on the allergen and how it enters the body, different people will experience various symptoms. Multiple body parts may simultaneously be affected by an allergic reaction.

Nose, eyes, sinuses, and throat

When an allergen is inhaled, histamine is released, causing the nasal lining to secrete more mucus and swell and irritate. It makes the nose run, itches, and may even cause violent sneezing. A sore throat and watery eyes are possible side effects.

chest and the lungs

During an allergic reaction, asthma may be brought on.

Breathing becomes challenging when an allergen is inhaled because the lining of the lungs' passages swells.

Abdomen and bowel

Peanuts, seafood, dairy, and eggs are among the foods that frequently cause allergies. Infants may develop a cow's milk allergy, which can result in eczema, asthma, colic, and stomach discomfort.

Lactose, the milk sugar, is indigestible for some people.

Stomach discomfort is a symptom of lactose intolerance, which is distinct from an allergy.

Skin

Urticaria (hives) and atopic dermatitis (eczema), two skin conditions that can be brought on by allergies.

Allergies that pose a serious risk to one's life must be treated right away.

Most allergic reactions are mild to moderate in intensity and don't result in significant issues. Anaphylaxis, a severe allergic reaction that necessitates immediate life-saving medication, can happen to a small percentage of people. Food, insect, and medication allergies are all potential anaphylaxis triggers. A severe allergy sufferer should have an ASCIA Action Plan for Anaphylaxis.

Options for treatment and prevention that work are available

Identification of the allergen's cause and mitigation of exposure to the allergen are essential components of allergen avoidance or minimization. People who are allergic to mites, for instance, may find that fewer dust mites in the home help to lessen their symptoms.

These drugs are some of those used to treat allergies

Antihistamines prevent mast cells from releasing histamine, which lessens symptoms. Antihistamine tablets without sedation are sold by pharmacies without a prescription. Other options include the use of antihistamine nasal and eye sprays.

When administered properly, intranasal corticosteroid nasal sprays (INCS) are effective in treating mild to severe allergic rhinitis.

Stronger doses of INCS might need a prescription.

Consult your physician or pharmacist for recommendations.

In order to benefit from the benefits of both drugs, combination therapies (INCS and antihistamine) are used to treat moderate to severe allergic rhinitis.

Ask your doctor or pharmacist for advice if you think using medicated eye drops will help you.

Epinephrine, also known as adrenaline, is used to treat anaphylaxis, which is a serious allergic reaction that can be fatal. With an adrenaline autoinjector, which can be administered without medical training, adrenaline is typically administered.

Sinusitis and allergic rhinitis can be treated without medication using saline sprays.

A long-term therapy called allergen immunotherapy, also referred to as desensitization, modifies how the immune system reacts to allergens. It entails giving regular, gradually increasing doses of allergen extracts via injections, as well as via sublingual tablets, sprays, or drops.

Allergies: What Are They?

When your body's natural defenses react to a foreign substance that is not harmful to the body, allergies can develop. These include things like pollen, dust, and particular foods. Histamine is released when your immune system recognizes these substances. A reaction to an allergen is brought on by histamine.

Which Things Typically Set Off Allergies?

A variety of substances, such as:

- Pollen.

- a dust mite.

- Mold.

- Pet hair.

- Various foods (e.g.,dairy products, and shellfish).

What Are the Advantages of Natural Allergy Treatments?

Due to the potential for fewer side effects than prescription medications, many people choose natural remedies for allergies. Natural cures may also be more affordable and available to some people.

The Homeopathic Treatments for Allergies

Many natural remedies are used by people to treat allergies and reduce their symptoms. Even though not all natural treatments for allergies are effective for everyone, some of the most well-liked choices include the following:

Regional honey

For its medicinal qualities, local honey has been used for centuries. According to research, regularly consuming local honey (at a high dose) can help lessen allergy symptoms since it may contain trace amounts of pollen.

Probiotics

Live bacteria and yeasts are considered probiotics. They are healthy for you, particularly for your digestive system. Probiotics may help people who have allergy symptoms live longer, according to some studies.

vitamins C

Antioxidant qualities of vitamin C shield cells from harm. According to studies conducted by the National Institute of Health, intravenous vitamin C may help lessen allergy symptoms. According to the study, vitamin C benefits patients with allergic diseases by reducing oxidative stress and inflammation.

Quercetin

Apples, onions, and berries are just a few examples of the foods that contain the plant pigment quercetin. Quercetin supplementation may help lessen allergy symptoms, according to research. The antioxidant and anti-inflammatory properties of quercetin are strong. It is excellent for treating allergic reactions due to its anti-allergic mechanism of action, which involves inhibiting enzymes and inflammatory mediators.

Leaf of a nettle

Natural antihistamines and anti-inflammatory herbs, such as nettle leaf, are used to treat allergies.

According to the sino-nasal outcome test (SNOT-22), nettle leaves may be effective in treating allergies, as some studies have suggested.

Butterbur

For its medicinal benefits, the plant butterbur has been used for centuries.

According to some studies, butterbur extracts can lessen the symptoms of hay fever and other allergies.

Butterbur has similar effects to cetirizine, according to research.

Acupuncture

In traditional Chinese medicine, acupuncture is used to treat allergies.

At specific locations on the body, needles are inserted into the skin.

According to studies, acupuncture's regulation of the cytokine profile may help to lessen allergic reactions.

Rinsing the nose

Using a saline solution, one performs nasal rinsing to clean the nasal passages. Congestion and other allergy symptoms may be lessened by doing this. It effectively clears allergens and irritants from your nasal passages.

vinegar made from apple juice

Atopic dermatitis sufferers in particular have reported fewer allergy symptoms after using apple cider vinegar, according to medical professionals. Apply the mixture to the affected area after mixing one cup of warm water and one tablespoon of apple cider vinegar. For best results, leave overnight.

A specialist in allergies should still be consulted

Overall, for some people, natural remedies can be a beneficial addition to allergy treatment.

They often lessen allergy symptoms, according to many people.

However, different people may experience different levels of success with different treatments. You should consult your doctor to make sure a natural allergy remedy is safe before trying it. Remember that the use of these remedies should never be used in place of medical care.

The best course of treatment for your allergies should be decided by your allergist.

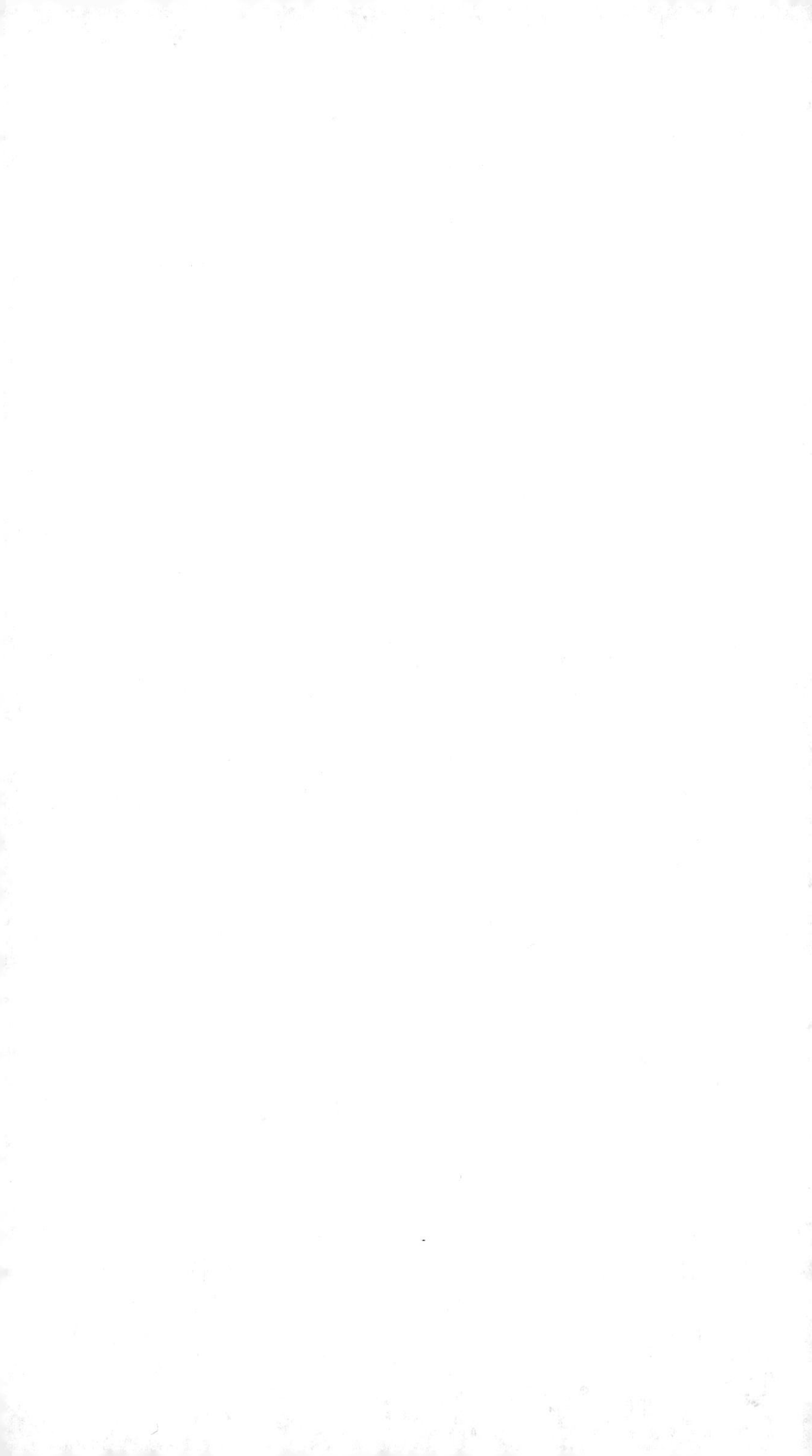

www.ingramcontent.com/pod-product-compliance
Lightning Source LLC
Chambersburg PA
CBHW070804260726
48660CB00005B/1697